Cambridge Elements ⁼

Elements in Molecular Oncology
edited by
Edward P. Gelmann
University of Arizona

PERSONALIZED DRUG SCREENING FOR FUNCTIONAL TUMOR PROFILING

Victoria El-Khoury
Luxembourg Institute of Health

Tatiana Michel
Luxembourg Institute of Health

Hichul Kim
Luxembourg Institute of Health

Yong-Jun Kwon
Luxembourg Institute of Health

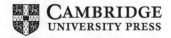
CAMBRIDGE
UNIVERSITY PRESS

CAMBRIDGE
UNIVERSITY PRESS

University Printing House, Cambridge CB2 8BS, United Kingdom

One Liberty Plaza, 20th Floor, New York, NY 10006, USA

477 Williamstown Road, Port Melbourne, VIC 3207, Australia

314–321, 3rd Floor, Plot 3, Splendor Forum, Jasola District Centre,
New Delhi – 110025, India

103 Penang Road, #05–06/07, Visioncrest Commercial, Singapore 238467

Cambridge University Press is part of the University of Cambridge.

It furthers the University's mission by disseminating knowledge in the pursuit of
education, learning, and research at the highest international levels of excellence.

www.cambridge.org
Information on this title: www.cambridge.org/9781009016933
DOI: 10.1017/9781009037877

First published 2022

A catalogue record for this publication is available from the British Library.

ISBN 978-1-009-01693-3 Paperback
ISSN 2634-7490 (online)
ISSN 2634-7482 (print)

Cambridge University Press has no responsibility for the persistence or accuracy of
URLs for external or third-party internet websites referred to in this publication
and does not guarantee that any content on such websites is, or will remain,
accurate or appropriate.

Every effort has been made in preparing this Element to provide accurate and
up-to-date information which is in accord with accepted standards and practice at the
time of publication. Although case histories are drawn from actual cases, every effort
has been made to disguise the identities of the individuals involved. Nevertheless, the
authors, editors and publishers can make no warranties that the information
contained herein is totally free from error, not least because clinical standards are
constantly changing through research and regulation. The authors, editors and
publishers therefore disclaim all liability for direct or consequential damages resulting
from the use of material contained in this book. Readers are strongly advised to pay
careful attention to information provided by the manufacturer of any drugs or
equipment that they plan to use.

Personalized Drug Screening for Functional Tumor Profiling

Elements in Molecular Oncology

DOI: 10.1017/9781009037877
First published online: June 2022

Victoria El-Khoury
Luxembourg Institute of Health

Tatiana Michel
Luxembourg Institute of Health

Hichul Kim
Luxembourg Institute of Health

Yong-Jun Kwon
Luxembourg Institute of Health

Author for correspondence: Victoria El-Khoury, Victoria.ElKhoury@lih.lu

Abstract: Despite considerable advances in our understanding of the biology that underlies tumor development and progression of cancer and the rapidly evolving field of personalized medicine, cancer is still one of the deadliest diseases. Many cancer patients have benefited from the survival improvements observed with targeted therapies but only a small subset of patients receiving targeted drugs experience an objective response. Because cancer is a complex and heterogeneous disease, the search for effective cancer treatments will need to address not only patient-specific molecular defects but also aspects of the tumor microenvironment. The functional tumor profiling directly measures the cellular phenotype, in particular tumor growth, in response to drugs using patient-derived tumor models and might be the next step toward precision oncology. In this Element, the authors discuss the personalized drug screening as a novel patient stratification strategy for the determination of individualized treatment choices in oncology.

Keywords: targeted therapy, personalized medicine, precision medicine, drug screening, personalized functional profiling

ISBNs: 9781009016933 (PB), 9781009037877 (OC)
ISSNs: 2634-7490 (online), 2634-7482 (print)

Contents

1 Rationale for Functional Profiling in Oncology

Cancer is the second leading cause of death worldwide. In 2020, the estimated numbers of new cases of invasive cancer and related death in the USA exceed 1.8 million and 606,000, respectively [1]. Since 1991, the cancer mortality rate has declined continuously in the USA, reaching an overall drop of 29% since 2017. The decline in cancer-related mortality is mainly attributed both to changes in smoking habits and to recent treatment advances. Nevertheless, the incidence of some cancers continues to rise, as is the case for cancers of the pancreas, liver and thyroid, while progress in treatment options is slowing for cancers amenable to early detection [1]. In addition, many cancer patients with advanced disease do not benefit from robust therapeutic options [2]; therefore, the development of effective anticancer treatment strategies is still an urgent medical need.

Over the last decade, molecular diagnostics has considerably promoted precision medicine in cancer through the identification of specific actionable mutations [3]. One of the first successes of precision medicine in solid tumor oncology was the discovery that a subset of non-small cell lung cancer (NSCLC) patients harboring specific somatic mutations in the epidermal growth factor receptor (EGFR) gene have a marked therapeutic response to EGFR tyrosine kinase inhibitors (EGFR TKIs) [4,5]. Although the majority of cancer patients have at least one molecular alteration, the percentage of advanced patients that have actionable alterations varies from approximately 10% to more than 50%, depending on the study cohort [2,6]. However, only a small subset of advanced cancer patients (13%) receiving molecular-targeted drugs experience an objective response [6]. Integrating tumor molecular markers, mainly genomic data, with functional profiling, namely, drug screening, will undoubtedly increase the therapeutic options and impact treatment outcomes. Ideally, personalized drug screening is performed with primary patient samples to provide rapidly efficient drugs with low toxicity.

In the first drug screening programs, initiated, among others, by Memorial Sloan Kettering in the 1940s, mouse models were used for screening potential anticancer agents [7]. In 1976, the Division of Cancer Treatment and Diagnosis (DCTD) of the National Cancer Institute (NCI) incorporated the use of human colon, breast and lung tumor xenograft models in the primary screening program of the Cancer Chemotherapy National Service Center (CCNSC). However, until the beginning of the 1980s, all of the molecules used in a drug screen were first evaluated in mouse leukemia models, leading to discovery of only a paucity of drugs as effective against solid cancers. This prompted the NCI to develop a screening program using human tumor cell lines [7].

It involved the application of two-dimensional (2D) culture conditions that helped identify some promising drug combinations, leading to new clinical trials [8]. However, only 5–7% of anticancer drugs developed from standard cell line screens in conventional 2D culture demonstrated success in clinical trials [9,10], and only 3.4% of phase I–III clinical trials investigating these anticancer compounds had degrees of success [11]. Considering the duration and cost of anticancer drug development, the low success rate of preclinical compounds in clinical trials calls for the use of more structurally relevant tumor models in drug screening to achieve a more reliable prediction of drug efficacy and toxicity.

The concept of patient-specific drug sensitivity was proposed decades ago. Hamburger and Salmon were among the first to propose an in vitro drug sensitivity test of anticancer agents for patient treatment [12]. Their work was based on studies carried out at the Ontario Cancer Institute in Toronto in the 1960s and early 1970s that showed the possibility of assessing the growth and chemosensitivity of some murine tumors in vitro using colony-forming assays in a semisolid medium [13,14]. Hamburger and Salmon developed this system at the University of Arizona Cancer Center to support the growth of human tumor cells [15,16]. In the mid-1970s, they proposed the human tumor colony-forming assay (HTCA) and tested it on samples from patients with multiple myeloma and various solid tumors [12,16,17]. This test has provided clear evidence of patient-to-patient heterogeneity in drug sensitivity and of its capacity to predict response to treatment [12,18,19]. In particular, in 1978, Salmon et al. reported their first results of correlation between in vitro chemosensitivity and in vivo tumor response of nine multiple myeloma patients and nine ovarian carcinoma patients. They observed a high correlation between in vitro drug resistance and a lack of clinical response, and some degree of concordance between in vitro and in vivo chemosensitivity [12]. In a retrospective study on 123 cancer patients, the HTCA displayed very good positive (0.88) and negative (0.94) predictive values when comparing the in vitro results of the test and the clinical responses [20]. These data are in line with other reports demonstrating that the HTCA could accurately predict drug resistance and, to a lesser extent, drug sensitivity [12,19,21–24]. Overall, the HTCA results suggest a 60–80% chance of clinical response if the patients are treated with a drug that inhibits colony formation in vitro. This percentage drops to 5–15% if the drug does not display an activity in the HTCA [25]. Von Hoff et al. compared the clinical outcome of patients with advanced malignancies after receiving a treatment selected empirically by the clinician or based on the results of a modified cloning assay. They observed that the partial response rate for the patients who received a test-directed individual therapy was significantly higher than the rate for patients who received the treatment selected empirically by the clinician (21% versus 3%) [26]. However, while improving the response rate, the in vitro drug sensitivity assay did not improve patients' survival [26, 27]. Importantly, the feasibility of the HTCA was dependent on the ability of primary tumors to form colonies in soft agar. Unfortunately, not all tumors formed colonies in vitro, and the cloning efficiency (i.e. the number of colonies formed/number of cells plated) in this system was very low, ranging from 0.01% to 0.1% for many tumor types. These technical limitations combined with the scarcity of tumor cells in some clinical specimens resulted in the applicability of the HTCA for only 25% of cancer patients [19,20]. Nevertheless, for many years, the HTCA proved more predictive of an individual tumor's responsiveness to anticancer agents than other newly developed in vitro drug sensitivity tests, such as the radiometric system [28]. The HTCA was adopted by different research laboratories and laid the foundation for the development of improved drug sensitivity assays [24,26,29–32].

2 Tumor Models in Drug Screening

2.1 Two-Dimensional versus Three-Dimensional Cultures

The 2D cell culture is a simple, reproducible, convenient, rapid and cost-effective method for screening a large number of compounds. This system has significantly contributed to our understanding of cell behavior and drugs' mechanisms of action. However, it is becoming evident that 2D cell cultures cannot always accurately select clinically active molecules. They fail to mimic the three-dimensional (3D) tissue architecture, thus affecting, among others, the treatment response. Cancer cells are not the only determinants of a tumor's characteristics and behavior in vivo [33]. The tumor microenvironment (TME), namely the extracellular matrix (ECM), consisting of a network of proteins and proteoglycans, and the cellular components including, but not limited to, stromal fibroblasts, endothelial cells and immune cells, are key factors in cancer progression, metastasis and drug resistance [34,35]. Initial studies in ovarian cancer showed that cells cultured as aggregates are less sensitive to drugs than monolayer cell cultures [36,37]. Similarly, breast cancer cell lines cultured as multicellular spheroids were more resistant to paclitaxel and doxorubicin than the same cells grown in 2D conditions [38]. Further studies comparing the 2D and 3D cultures of colorectal cancer (CRC) cells revealed differences in signaling pathways and drug responses and showed that 3D cultures faithfully recapitulate the in vivo situation [39]. Many signaling pathways involved in chemoresponsiveness are differentially activated in monolayer cultures, which results in 2D cultures that are often (but not always) more sensitive to drug therapies, leading to false-positive screening data [37]. Evidence has been provided to support the idea that efficacy and toxicity of drugs tested in 3D models match clinical data [40,41]. These findings suggest that the format of the cell culture shapes cellular drug responses and affects the translational potential of a molecule [42]. Indeed, 2D cell cultures do not recapitulate the gradients of drugs, nutrients, gases and waste products that characterize tumors in vivo; all are important factors that influence response to therapy [43,44]. Cells in 2D culture are forced to adopt a sheet-like morphology that does not reflect the real structural organization of the cells in vivo, as is the case for the monolayer propagation of pancreatic ductal adenocarcinoma cell lines in 2D cultures while they are polarized and well-organized structures in vivo [45]. Hepatocytes are another example of cells whose physiology is considerably affected by culture conditions. Hepatocytes are characterized by a multipolar organization and their dedifferentiation in 2D cell cultures alters major liver functions, namely detoxification and production of plasma proteins [46]. Also, the cancer cell monolayer culture reduces the deposition of the ECM, an active contributor to tumor progression, cancer phenotype and gene expression [47]. As a consequence, drugs that act on the ECM to kill cancer cells cannot be accurately evaluated under monolayer cell culture conditions [35]. An alternative and necessary approach for drug testing is to use preclinical 3D models capable of restoring the architecture of solid tumors, by retaining cell–cell and cell–matrix interactions. The patient-derived tumor xenograft (PDX) model has become one of the most important platforms for in vivo preclinical research in personalized medicine and drug screening. Several ex vivo models used in 3D cell cultures have also demonstrated the ability to recapitulate the patient's tumor characteristics. An important advantage of 3D cell culture is that it eliminates the contribution to the observed outcomes of factors inherent to the host (animal models), and thus allows drug testing directly in relevant human models. Different 3D cell culture techniques exist but not all are compatible with high-throughput screening [48].

2.2 Patient-Derived Tumor Xenograft (PDX) Models

Patient-derived tumor xenograft models have emerged to be among the most exciting and useful models for cancer precision medicine. These models are established by engrafting patient tumor tissues into host animals, most commonly immunocompromised mice [49]. The PDX models retain many of the characteristics of the original patient's tumor, including histology, genomic profile, growth potential, heterogeneity and drug responsiveness [49–51]. In the 1980s, studies on lung cancer and childhood rhabdomyosarcoma revealed the high correlation between response to treatment in clinic and in PDX models [52,53].

In the last decade, PDX models have been successfully applied to assess response to therapy and discovery or validation of biomarkers in many cancer types [50,54,55]. Interestingly, xenograft models identified a synergism between vincristine and topotecan, a combination currently used in the treatment of some childhood solid cancers [56]. These models have also shown the effectiveness of the combination of nab-paclitaxel and gemcitabine in pancreatic ductal adenocarcinoma, results that correlated with the clinical efficacy of this association [57,58]. They are especially advantageous for improving clinical trial design [50]. For example, preclinical evaluation of new agents on PDX models with known histologic, molecular and genomic profiles may validate a genetically based hypothesis, reveal resistance mechanisms or help select the population of patients that will most likely be responsive to the drug [50,59]. In order to foster translational cancer research, several academic and industrial groups have developed PDX biorepositories as tools for drug development and biomarker screening. The Novartis Institutes for BioMedical Research PDX encyclopedia (NIBR PDXE) is an example of a collection of 1,075 PDX models with well-characterized genomic profiles that was successfully used for biomarker identification and validation and for the prediction of population-based clinical trial drug response in high-throughput screening [60]. Other large PDX collections in the USA include the NCI repository of patient-derived models (PDMR), the Public Repository of Xenografts (PRoXe) developed by the Weinstock Laboratory at Dana–Farber Cancer Institute [61] and the Jackson Laboratory PDX cohort [62]. A European initiative began in 2013 was known as EurOPDX, a consortium of cancer centers and universities (18 members so far) that has established PDX collections (~1,500 PDX models in total), in order to promote collaborative scientific projects and multicenter preclinical trials [50]. Patient-derived tumor xenograft models are also used as a preclinical personalized medicine platform to guide patient therapy. Indeed, with their ability to predict clinical outcome, PDX models can serve as patient "avatars" for drug testing in coclinical trials where drug responses in mice are explored to choose the therapy to be administered to the patient [63,64]. For example, studies at Johns Hopkins University School of Medicine demonstrated the potential of PDX models to guide treatment decision-making for patients with advanced cancers [55,65], which prompted the creation of Champions Oncology in 2007, a company that provides translational oncology services using personalized "TumorGrafts®" – that is, murine avatars.

Patient-derived tumor xenograft models, and in particular avatar mouse models, will definitely continue to contribute in advancing precision cancer therapeutics. However, they face several challenges for routine use in personalized medicine: In addition to the variable engraftment success rate of the PDX models [51] and the length of time required for a successful implantation and propagation of the tumor (several months) [51,63], the results obtained with PDX models may be affected by the unavoidable effects of murine stromal components, the possible generation of false-positive and false-negative responses due to the different pharmacokinetics and toxicity of some drugs in mice and in humans [66], and the necessity of using immunocompromised mice that hampers any study targeting the immune system [45,63]. The emergence of immunocompetent "humanized" mice have the potential to compensate for the lack of immune system in PDX models; however, these models also face several limitations (i.e. lengthy procedures and hurdles to achieve a faithful reconstitution of human immune system, etc.) and their use for cancer research is still being demonstrated [67]. Other nonnegligible constraints in animal models are the cost, resources and logistics associated with their maintenance. In order to select the most efficient treatment for a particular patient, an alternative to the avatar strategy is the use of other 3D personalized models, such as organotypic tumor slices, spheroids and organoids.

2.3 Organotypic Tumor Slices

Organotypic tumor slices are a 3D representation of the tumor that faithfully preserve the complexity and the morphology of the tissue in vivo, in that the tumor cells are not removed from their original microenvironment through tissue dissociation; the tissue is rather cut in thin slices (250–500 μm) using a specifically designed device, most often a vibratome, and cultured freely floating in the medium or on a membrane [68,69]. Organotypic tumor slices from lung, prostate, colon, gastric, esophagogastric junction, breast, brain, and head and neck cancers were successfully established and used for assessing the drug sensitivity of the tumors [5,68–71]. They could also predict cytotoxic responses ex vivo [72]. Interestingly, tumor slices appeared to be effective models to test cytotoxic drugs and targeted therapies, including immunomodulatory agents [73]. The main disadvantage of this model in drug testing is its use in a relatively low-throughput setting because of poor cell propagation due to cell viability issues when tumor slices are cultured for extended periods [68]. Optimization of media composition and culture conditions (e.g. culturing under rotational movements or on Teflon membrane inserts) improved the preservation of tumor slices for up to 7 days in culture [72]. The readout of a drug screen using tumor slices is an additional drawback of this model. In fact, contrarily to other 3D models, the markers generally used in tissue slices for determining drug response are analyzed by immunoassays after tissue fixation, which can be technically laborious, requires special equipment and may introduce some quantification challenges [68]. Nevertheless, in addition to the faithful representation of the tumor in its microenvironment, the tumor slices have the advantage of being quickly generated and providing drug screening results within days, a time frame compatible with the clinical management of cancer. In conclusion, organotypic tumor slices represent a physiologically relevant 3D model for evaluating and predicting drug efficacy in a low-throughput test and hold great potential in improving personalized medicine. Patient-derived tumor spheroids and organoids in monoculture or coculture with stromal and/or immune cells remain the major 3D tools used in high- and medium-throughput drug screens for personalized cancer medicine.

2.4 Patient-Derived Tumor Spheroids and Organoids

The terms "spheroid" and "organoid" are often used interchangeably but there are main differences between them that need to be highlighted. Briefly, patient-derived tumor spheroids are obtained from tumor tissue incompletely digested into small multicellular entities that self-assemble and aggregate in a 3D tissue "micro" architecture. Patient-derived tumor organoids (PDOs) are grown from adult stem cells derived from the primary tumor. In general, PDOs are initiated by mechanical and enzymatic digestion into single cells and small fragments and cultured as self-organized 3D structures (resulting in a higher order structure, compared to spheroids) embedded in a 3D matrix (usually Matrigel) in the presence of essential growth factors and additional compounds to enhance cell viability and organoid passaging [74–76].

Patient-derived tumor organoids demonstrated high morphological and genetic similarity with the corresponding original tumors, as shown by the study of Weeber et al. that revealed that 90% of somatic mutations were shared between organoids and matching patients' tissues, and a correlation of 0.89 was observed in the DNA copy number profiles between both entities [77]. They were successfully used in proof-of-principle high-throughput drug screens that allowed the validation of gene–drug associations [2,78]. For example, tamoxifen was identified as a top scoring drug in an estrogen–receptor-positive (ER+) breast cancer patients' tumor cells. Also, drugs targeting the Raf/MEK/ERK pathway were selected from among more than 120 compounds as an effective treatment of a BRAF (V600E) mutant melanoma. The authors of the study were also able to nominate specific therapeutic options and identify unique combinations for individual patients, followed by their validation in vivo using PDX models [2]. Similarly, a proof-of-concept drug screen performed with 83 compounds in CRC organoids linked loss of p53 function to resistance to nutlin-3a, an E3 ubiquitin ligase (MDM2) inhibitor and mutation of *KRAS* was linked to resistance to EGFR inhibitors [78]. Drug screening trials using patient-derived tumor spheroids have also been reported. In this regard, 79 molecular-targeted agents were tested on patient-derived tumor spheroids from two endometrial cancer cases; the survivin inhibitor YM155 was identified as a hit drug and its cytotoxicity was subsequently assessed in spheroids from 11 endometrial cancer patients [79]. This small-scale proof-of-concept drug screen revealed the variable sensitivity of endometrial cancer cases to YM155. Interestingly, a high-throughput drug screen of 2,427 compounds was performed on two CRC patient-derived spheroids that were first expanded as mice xenografts and then dispensed into 384-well plates using an automated system; 15 compounds could be selected as hit drugs and were further evaluated in 30 CRC patient-derived spheroid lines [80].

3 Cell-Based Screening Platforms for Personalized Medicine

Cell-based high-throughput screening is a drug discovery approach to identify active compounds against a disease model. The high-throughput screening is integrated into a pipeline comprising a dispensing platform and imaging equipment to automate the process of drug screening and data acquisition. Until now, high-throughput screening has been used as a key tool for early drug development. In the last decade, there was a need to develop precision medicine for cancer patients. Now, high-throughput screening is being increasingly adopted in the development of personalized medicine. Several technologies have been tested to enable drug screening in physiologically relevant disease models.

3.1 Three-Dimensional Bioprinting Platform

Three-dimensional bioprinting is one of the most promising technologies expected to optimize the recapitulation of the disease complexity and thus the assessment of drug efficacy with improved physiological relevance and high reproducibility [81]. Three-dimensional culture systems and human tissue models are printed through a controlled and organized distribution of cells and active molecules on a surface, thus faithfully mimicking the tumor shape in vivo [81–84]. To generate a bioprinted model, spheroids are embedded into the appropriate tissue-like matrix such as Matrigel, collagen, alginate, synthetic peptides and polymers [85]. Three types of bioprinting have been developed, including droplet inkjet, microextrusion and laser-assisted bioprinting [86–88]. Datta et al. have recently summarized results with different 3D bioprinted cancer models for glioblastoma (GBM), breast cancer, pancreatic adenocarcinoma, ovarian cancer, cervical cancer and hepatocellular carcinoma [89–92]. The 3D bioprinted tumor model is suitable for predicting the response of tumor cells to an anticancer drug and allows the study of the mechanisms of drug response mediated by the microenvironment. It has been used as a platform for drug response in GBM [84,93] and cervical cancers [94].

Indeed, Yi et al. showed that the effects of radiotherapy and chemotherapy on a personalized GBM model were consistent with those actually seen in the respective patients, foreshadowing the development of personalized treatment schemes [84]. Using the cell printing technology, Zhao et al. generated HeLa cell spheroids in an alginate/gelatin/fibrinogen hydrogel, resulting in a cuboid structure with interconnected channels. The authors tested the resistance of the 3D printed constructs to paclitaxel by assessing cell morphology, metabolic activity and the distribution of spheroid diameters [94]. The 3D bioprinting technology holds great promise for the development of personalized therapeutics as patient-derived primary cells conserve the heterotypic composition of native tumor environment in the printed 3D model.

3.2 Micropillar-Based Cell Printing Platform

Different drug screening platforms based on nano- and micro-volume fluidics have been explored in the past decade to investigate the efficacy and toxicity of hundreds of drugs. Micropillar cell printing technology using 3D cell-based models is illustrated in Figure 1. This approach allows the screening of different drugs in clinical samples to identify the right drug for the patient in a personalized medicine approach. This technology is currently being tested by our group in a clinical trial (NCT03997617; https://clinicaltrials.gov/ct2/show/NCT03997617?cntry=LU&draw=3). The technology uses a micropillar and microwell/chip platform for high-throughput screening on in vitro 3D cell-based models from cancer patients [37,95]. The primary cells are encapsulated in alginate-based hydrogel drops and cultured in a micropillar chip, combined with a second microwell chip containing up to 60 different compounds of interest. Drugs are tested at different concentrations. Cell images are acquired using a high-content imaging instrument and image analysis software measures cell viability based on calcein AM fluorescence. The relative cell viability is obtained by normalizing each treatment condition with its corresponding control. Dose response curves (DRCs) are then generated, and the area under the DRC (AUC) and the half maximal inhibitory concentration (IC50) are calculated to quantify the efficacy of the drugs [37]. As few cells are needed from the patient and rapid, automated results can be achieved within a clinically practical time frame, these systems are particularly applicable for personalized medicine.

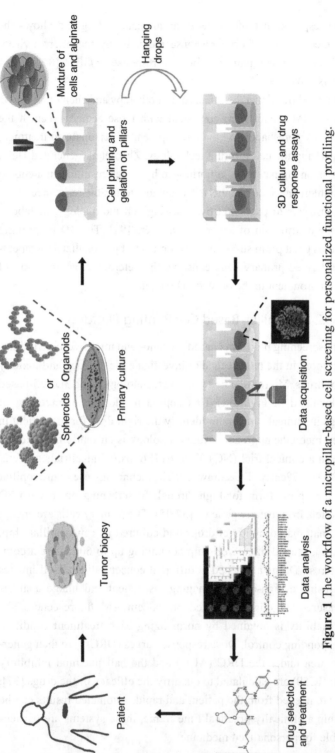

Figure 1 The workflow of a micropillar-based cell screening for personalized functional profiling.

4 Drug Repurposing in Personalized Oncomedicine

Drug libraries used in personalized drug screening contain either exclusively Food and Drug Administration (FDA)/European Medicines Agency (EMA)-approved drugs, or both approved and investigational drugs. The advantage of identifying an approved drug for a new indication is the starting points for drug repurposing, and may avoid the long approval process that characterizes drug development and the risk of prohibitive safety issues that may arise. Therefore, identifying a known drug for a new purpose may quickly trigger the "bedside-to-bench-to-bedside" cycle, provided that it is the same administration route as the original indication employed [96,97]. In general, drug repurposing integrates data from systems biology, including wet-lab experiments and computational approaches, in vitro screens of approved drug libraries, synthetic chemistry, in vivo phenotypic studies using human cells, and most importantly clinical trials [97,98]. Using this approach, several well-known noncancer drugs were repositioned for cancer treatments or were selected as drug-repurposing candidates for cancer prevention and/or treatment. For example, thalidomide, previously used as a sedative drug and to relieve pregnancy nausea and then withdrawn from the market due to teratogenicity, is now repositioned for refractory multiple myeloma. Evidence obtained from in vitro studies, preclinical and clinical studies, suggested the potential of metformin, a hypoglycemic drug, in cancer prevention [99]. Similarly, based on clinical data, the anti-inflammatory drug acetylsalicylic acid (aspirin) and other cyclooxygenase-2 inhibitors were shown to decrease the risk of CRC incidence and recurrence [98]. In oncology, individualized drug repurposing screens can be used to find rapidly an efficient treatment to a patient using the patient's own tumor cells. In this regard, it is important to select those patients who would benefit the most from personalized drug screening due to lack of available treatments for their disease or patients receiving inefficient or detrimental therapy. An interesting example of a drug repurposing was performed on cultures derived from tumor samples of a patient suffering from a recurrent respiratory papillomatosis [100]. The standard treatment of this generally benign tumor is surgery. However, when papillomatosis extends into the lung, there are no effective therapies and the tumor is almost always fatal. In a case report, lung tumor and normal adjacent tissues from a patient with chemoresistant progressive disease were processed into single cells and propagated as patient-derived cell cultures [100]. Genomic analysis of the sample revealed a mutated human papillomavirus (HPV)-11 genome. Of three candidate drugs – cidofovir used for treating the recurrent respiratory papillomatosis, dihydroartemisinin and vorinostat, both known to be effective in HPV-positive cancer cell lines – vorinostat was selected based on the drug screen and was used successfully for patient treatment [100]. Personalized drug repurposing screens were also useful in identifying effective drugs in GBM. From a library of 4,000 approved drugs and bioactive molecules, Gorshkov et al. conducted individualized drug screens on patient-derived tumor cells from four different GBM patients. The primary hit compounds were then tested in cells from seven patient samples and showed variable activities among the samples. Also, some patient samples displayed a profile compatible with increased sensitivity to chemotherapy when compared to other patient samples [96].

The search for existing drugs to target main cancer regulators has prompted the development of several algorithms to try to capture the complexity of the disease. While most of these algorithms failed to fulfill this objective and hence could not move to the clinic, the VIPER (Virtual Inference of Protein Activity by Enriched Regulon analysis) algorithm, developed by Alvarez and Califano at Columbia University, is a clear breakthrough in the field of computational modeling [101]. Califano's approach is based on the analysis of whole transcriptome sequencing of a given tumor sample to infer aberrant protein activity and thus elucidate the available compounds that target these "master regulator proteins" [102,103]. In 2015, Califano and Bosker founded DarwinHealth, a Manhattan-based biotechnology company, and applied VIPER technology to patients' specimens [104]. An initial trial analyzing up to 3,000 cancer patients with DarwinHealth algorithms demonstrated a high therapeutic response-predictive potential of DarwinHealth approach [104,105]. Two precision medicine tests, Darwin OncoTarget^{TM} and Darwin OncoTreat^{TM}, developed by DarwinHealth, in 2018 received the approval of the New York State Department of Health and are already used in many clinical trials around the world to guide the treatment of cancer patients [104]. This novel precision oncology platform will undoubtedly complement the drug screening approach to improve personalized cancer therapies and to foster drug repurposing.

5 Clinical Applications of Drug Screening in Oncology

Several clinical trials are currently in place to assess the feasibility and usefulness of functional tumor profiling in cancer management and treatment. A large multicenter cohort study (TUMOROID trial, NL49002.031.14) was initiated by Utrecht University in the Netherlands to determine if organoids can predict treatment response of patients with metastatic CRC, breast cancer or NSCLC. Whereas the TUMOROID trial evaluated if PDO can recapitulate tumor drug sensitivity in the patient, the SENSOR (NL50400.031.14) clinical study was launched to guide treatment choice. To do so, a small-scale screening of eight different targeted molecules is performed on patient organoids from metastatic CRC and NSCLC before they start their last standard-of-care treatment. If one of the treatments is active in vitro, the patient is offered the targeted therapy [106].

Our group has recently launched a pilot study (NCT03997617) to evaluate the clinical feasibility of integrated personalized functional profiling for patients with metastatic gastrointestinal cancer or recurrent GBM. This study includes screening of patient-derived tumor spheroids with FDA/EMA-approved drugs and issuing treatment recommendation to the clinician who will decide whether or not to follow this recommendation.

Whereas the use of adjuvant chemotherapy in stage IA NSCLC tumors after curative resection (R0) is not recommended, it remains unclear how to treat a relapsed tumor of a resected early-stage NSCLC. Interestingly, five EGFR-targeted TKIs were tested on organoids established from a lymph node metastasis of a lung adenocarcinoma, following recurrence of a stage IA1 tumor harboring EGFR L858R and TP53 R110L mutations after R0 resection. Based on the results of the DRCs, osimertinib was selected and administered to the patient who achieved a progression-free survival of 9 months [107].

6 Conclusions and Perspectives

The concept of functional tumor profiling is emerging as a promising approach to predict treatment efficacy and to determine the best treatment for individual cancer patients. Whereas genomics can identify a plausible effective approved targeted therapy, personalized drug screening may refine treatment options by assessing several drug combinations and testing novel investigational molecules drugs for off-label use. Screening should prioritize drugs that match the cancer profile – for instance, molecules that target identified cancer mutations in the original tumor – and should be performed at clinically relevant concentrations. An integrative approach combining clinical, genomic and response data generated from hundreds to thousands of samples will help prioritize the drugs to include in a personalized drug screen. Future research should address the challenges of functional drug profiling, mainly (1) improving the generation of personalized humanized mouse models (where tumor and immune system are from the same patient) for personalized drug screening; (2) optimizing the establishment of 3D models using limited amounts of tissue; (3) developing 3D cell cultures from circulating tumor cells in body fluids, including blood, ascites and pleural effusion; (4) improving the coculture approaches with tumor cells and cells from the microenvironment; and (5) optimizing the culture and drug screening conditions in order to deliver meaningful results back to the clinic within acceptable time frames, ideally measured as days to a few weeks.

References

1. RL Siegel, KD Miller and A Jemal: Cancer statistics, 2020. CA Cancer J. Clin. 70: 7–30, 2020.

2. C Pauli, BD Hopkins, D Prandi et al.: Personalized in vitro and in vivo cancer models to guide precision medicine. Cancer Discov. 7:462–477, 2017.

3. CW Bennett, G Berchem, YJ Kim et al.: Cell-free DNA and next-generation sequencing in the service of personalized medicine for lung cancer. Oncotarget 7:71013–71035, 2016.

4. D Gonzalez de Castro, PA Clarke, B Al-Lazikani et al.: Personalized cancer medicine: Molecular diagnostics, predictive biomarkers, and drug resistance. Clin. Pharmacol. Ther. 93:252–259, 2013.

5. MM Gerlach, F Merz, G Wichmann et al.: Slice cultures from head and neck squamous cell carcinoma: A novel test system for drug susceptibility and mechanisms of resistance. Br. J. Cancer 110:479–488, 2014.

6. O Tredan, Q Wang, D Pissaloux et al.: Molecular screening program to select molecular-based recommended therapies for metastatic cancer patients: Analysis from the ProfiLER trial. Ann. Oncol. 30:757–765, 2019.

7. WR Waud: Murine L1210 and P388 leukemias, in Teicher B (ed.): Tumor Models in Cancer Research. Totowa, NJ, Humana Press, (2011, pp. 23–41.

8. SL Holbeck, R Camalier, JA Crowell et al.: The National Cancer Institute ALMANAC: A comprehensive screening resource for the detection of anticancer drug pairs with enhanced therapeutic activity. Cancer Res. 77:3564–3576, 2017.

9. M Hay, DW Thomas, JL Craighead et al.: Clinical development success rates for investigational drugs. Nat. Biotechnol. 32:40–51, 2014.

10. P Horvath, N Aulner, M Bickle et al.: Screening out irrelevant cell-based models of disease. Nat. Rev. Drug Discov. 15: 751–769, 2016.

11. CH Wong, KW Siah and AW Lo: Estimation of clinical trial success rates and related parameters. Biostatistics 20: 273–286, 2019.

12. SE Salmon, AW Hamburger, B Soehnlen et al.: Quantitation of differential sensitivity of human-tumor stem cells to anticancer drugs. N. Engl. J. Med. 298: 1321–1327, 1978.

13. WR Bruce, BE Meeker and FA Valeriote: Comparison of the sensitivity of normal hematopoietic and transplanted lymphoma colony-forming cells to chemotherapeutic agents administered in vivo. J. Natl. Cancer Inst. 37:233–245, 1966.

14. CH Park, DE Bergsagel and EA McCulloch: Mouse myeloma tumor stem cells: A primary cell culture assay. J. Natl. Cancer Inst. 46: 411–422, 1971.

15. SE Salmon: In vitro assay for sensitivity to anticancer drugs. Hosp. Pract. (Off. Ed.) 20:133–137, 141–142, 145–148, 1985.

16. AW Hamburger and SE Salmon: Primary bioassay of human tumor stem cells. Science 197:461–463, 1977.

17. A Hamburger and SE Salmon: Primary bioassay of human myeloma stem cells. J. Clin. Invest. 60:846–854, 1977.

18. DD von Hoff, GM Clark, BJ Stogdill et al.: Prospective clinical trial of a human tumor cloning system. Cancer Res. 43: 1926–1931, 1983.

19. SE Salmon: Human tumor colony assay and chemosensitivity testing. Cancer Treat. Rep. 68: 117–125, 1984.

20. DD vvon Hoff, J Casper, E Bradley et al.: Association between human tumor colony-forming assay results and response of an individual patient's tumor to chemotherapy. Am. J. Med. 70: 1027–1041, 1981.

21. BD Mann, DH Kern, AE Giuliano et al.: Clinical correlations with drug sensitivities in the clonogenic assay: A retrospective study. Arch. Surg. 117:33–36, 1982.

22. FL Meyskens, Jr., TE Moon, B Dana et al.: Quantitation of drug sensitivity by human metastatic melanoma colony-forming units. Br. J. Cancer 44:787–797, 1981.

23. DS Alberts, HS Chen, SE Salmon et al.: Chemotherapy of ovarian cancer directed by the human tumor stem cell assay. Cancer Chemother. Pharmacol. 6:279–285, 1981.

24. KH Link, M Kornmann, GH Leder et al.: Regional chemotherapy directed by individual chemosensitivity testing in vitro: A prospective decision-aiding trial. Clin. Cancer Res. 2: 1469–1474, 1996.

25. AR Hanauske, U Hanauske and DD von Hoff: Recent improvements in the human tumor cloning assay for sensitivity testing of antineoplastic agents. Eur. J. Cancer Clin. Oncol. 23:603–605, 1987.

26. DD von Hoff, JF Sandbach, GM Clark et al.: Selection of cancer chemotherapy for a patient by an in vitro assay versus a clinician. J. Natl. Cancer Inst. 82:110–116, 1990.

27. M Federico, DS Alberts, DJ Garcia et al.: In vitro drug testing of ovarian cancer using the human tumor colony-forming assay: Comparison of in vitro response and clinical outcome. Gynecol. Oncol. 55:S156–163, 1994.

28. DD von Hoff, BJ Forseth, JN Turner et al.: Selection of chemotherapy for patient treatment utilizing a radiometric versus a cloning system. Int.J. Cell Cloning 4:16–26, 1986.

29. DD von Hoff: Human tumor cloning assays: Applications in clinical oncology and new antineoplastic agent development. Cancer Metastasis Rev. 7: 357–371, 1988.

30. N Tanigawa, DH Kern, Y Hikasa et al.: Rapid assay for evaluating the chemosensitivity of human tumors in soft agar culture. Cancer Res. 42:2159–2164, 1982.

31. LM Weisenthal, JA Marsden, PL Dill et al.: A novel dye exclusion method for testing in vitro chemosensitivity of human tumors. Cancer Res. 43:749–757, 1983.

32. M Kornmann, U Butzer, J Blatter et al.: Pre-clinical evaluation of the activity of gemcitabine as a basis for regional chemotherapy of pancreatic and colorectal cancer. Eur. J. Surg. Oncol. 26:583–587, 2000.

33. KC Valkenburg, AE de Groot and KJ Pienta: Targeting the tumour stroma to improve cancer therapy. Nat. Rev. Clin. Oncol. 15: 366–381, 2018.

34. R Baghban, L Roshangar, R Jahanban-Esfahlan et al.: Tumor microenvironment complexity and therapeutic implications at a glance. Cell. Commun. Signal 18:59, 2020.

35. SC van der Steen, R Raave, S Langerak et al.: Targeting the extracellular matrix of ovarian cancer using functionalized, drug loaded lyophilisomes. Eur. J. Pharm. Biopharm. 113:229–239, 2017.

36. D Loessner, KS Stok, MP Lutolf et al.: Bioengineered 3D platform to explore cell-ECM interactions and drug resistance of epithelial ovarian cancer cells. Biomaterials 31:8494–8506, 2010.

37. DW Lee, YS Choi, YJ Seo et al.: High-throughput screening (HTS) of anticancer drug efficacy on a micropillar/microwell chip platform. Anal. Chem. 86:535–542, 2014.

38. Y Imamura, T Mukohara, Y Shimono et al.: Comparison of 2D- and 3D-culture models as drug-testing platforms in breast cancer. Oncol. Rep. 33: 1837–1843, 2015.

39. A Riedl, M Schlederer, K Pudelko et al.: Comparison of cancer cells in 2D vs 3D culture reveals differences in AKT-mTOR-S6 K signaling and drug responses. J. Cell. Sci. 130:203–218, 2017.

40. K Halfter, O Hoffmann, N Ditsch et al.: Testing chemotherapy efficacy in HER2 negative breast cancer using patient-derived spheroids. J. Transl. Med. 14:112, 2016.

41. P Gunness, D Mueller, V Shevchenko et al.: 3D organotypic cultures of human HepaRG cells: A tool for in vitro toxicity studies. Toxicol. Sci. 133:67–78, 2013.

42. J Jabs, FM Zickgraf, J Park et al.: Screening drug effects in patient-derived cancer cells links organoid responses to genome alterations. Mol. Syst. Biol. 13:955, 2017.

43. MD Hall, C Martin, DJ Ferguson et al.: Comparative efficacy of novel platinum(IV) compounds with established chemotherapeutic drugs in solid tumour models. Biochem. Pharmacol. 67:17–30, 2004.

44. RM Sutherland: Cell and environment interactions in tumor microregions: The multicell spheroid model. Science 240: 177–184, 1988.

45. CI Hwang, SF Boj, H Clevers et al.: Preclinical models of pancreatic ductal adenocarcinoma. J. Pathol. 238:197–204, 2016.

46. P Godoy, NJ Hewitt, U Albrecht et al.: Recent advances in 2D and 3D in vitro systems using primary hepatocytes, alternative hepatocyte sources and non-parenchymal liver cells and their use in investigating mechanisms of hepatotoxicity, cell signaling and ADME. Arch. Toxicol. 87: 1315–1530, 2013.

47. XZ Wu, D Chen and GR Xie: Extracellular matrix remodeling in hepatocellular carcinoma: Effects of soil on seed? Med. Hypotheses 66: 1115–1120, 2006.

48. Y Fang and RM Eglen: Three-dimensional cell cultures in drug discovery and development. SLAS Discov. 22: 456–472, 2017.

49. JJ Tentler, AC Tan, CD Weekes et al.: Patient-derived tumour xenografts as models for oncology drug development. Nat. Rev. Clin. Oncol. 9:338–350, 2012.

50. M Hidalgo, F Amant, AV Biankin et al.: Patient-derived xenograft models: An emerging platform for translational cancer research. Cancer Discov. 4:998–1013, 2014.

51. SY Cho: Patient-derived xenografts as compatible models for precision oncology. Lab. Anim. Res. 36: 14, 2020.

52. JA Houghton, PJ Houghton and AA Green: Chemotherapy of childhood rhabdomyosarcomas growing as xenografts in immune-deprived mice. Cancer Res. 42:535–539, 1982.

53. HH Fiebig, HA Neumann, H Henss et al.: Development of three human small cell lung cancer models in nude mice. Recent Results Cancer Res. 97:77–86, 1985.

54. E Rosfjord, J Lucas, G Li et al.: Advances in patient-derived tumor xenografts: From target identification to predicting clinical response rates in oncology. Biochem. Pharmacol. 91:135–143, 2014.

55. M Hidalgo, E Bruckheimer, NV Rajeshkumar et al.: A pilot clinical study of treatment guided by personalized tumorgrafts in patients with advanced cancer. Mol. Cancer Ther. 10: 1311–1316, 2011.

56. J Thompson, EO George, CA Poquette et al.: Synergy of topotecan in combination with vincristine for treatment of pediatric solid tumor xenografts Clin. Cancer Res. 5:3617–3631, 1999s.

57. DD von Hoff, RK Ramanathan, MJ Borad et al.: Gemcitabine plus nab-paclitaxel is an active regimen in patients with advanced pancreatic cancer: A phase I/II trial. J. Clin. Oncol. 29: 4548–4554, 2011.

58. DD von Hoff, T Ervin, FP Arena et al.: Increased survival in pancreatic cancer with nab-paclitaxel plus gemcitabine. N. Engl. J. Med. 369: 1691–1703, 2013.

59. MR Girotti, F Lopes, N Preece et al.: Paradox-breaking RAF inhibitors that also target SRC are effective in drug-resistant BRAF mutant melanoma. Cancer Cell 27:85–96, 2015.

60. H Gao, JM Korn, S Ferretti et al.: High-throughput screening using patient-derived tumor xenografts to predict clinical trial drug response. Nat. Med. 21: 1318–1325, 2015.

61. EC Townsend, MA Murakami, A Christodoulou et al.: The Public Repository of Xenografts enables discovery and randomized phase II-like trials in mice. Cancer Cell 29:574–586, 2016.

62. T Goto: Patient-derived tumor xenograft models: Toward the establishment of precision cancer medicine. J. Pers. Med. 10: 64, 2020.

63. P Malaney, SV Nicosia and V Dave: One mouse, one patient paradigm: New avatars of personalized cancer therapy. Cancer Lett. 344:1–12, 2014.

64. JG Clohessy and PP Pandolfi: Mouse hospital and co-clinical trial project: From bench to bedside. Nat. Rev. Clin. Oncol. 12:491–498, 2015.

65. J Stebbing, K Paz, GK Schwartz et al.: Patient-derived xenografts for individualized care in advanced sarcoma. Cancer 120:2006–2015, 2014.

66. RT Kurmasheva and PJ Houghton: Identifying novel therapeutic agents using xenograft models of pediatric cancer. Cancer Chemother. Pharmacol. 78:221–232, 2016.

67. TM Allen, MA Brehm, S Bridges et al.: Humanized immune system mouse models: Progress, challenges and opportunities. Nat. Immunol. 20:770–774, 2019.

68. TG Meijer, KA Naipal, A Jager et al.: Ex vivo tumor culture systems for functional drug testing and therapy response prediction. Future Sci. OA 3: FSO190, 2017.

69. LF Horowitz, AD Rodriguez, Z Dereli-Korkut et al.: Multiplexed drug testing of tumor slices using a microfluidic platform. NPJ Precis. Oncol. 4:12, 2020.

70. J Koerfer, S Kallendrusch, F Merz et al.: Organotypic slice cultures of human gastric and esophagogastric junction cancer. Cancer Med. 5:1444–1453, 2016.

71. V Vaira, G Fedele, S Pyne et al.: Preclinical model of organotypic culture for pharmacodynamic profiling of human tumors. Proc. Natl. Acad. Sci. USA 107:8352–8356, 2010.

72. KA Naipal, NS Verkaik, H Sanchez et al.: Tumor slice culture system to assess drug response of primary breast cancer. BMC Cancer 16:78, 2016.

73. R Sivakumar, M Chan, JS Shin et al.: Organotypic tumor slice cultures provide a versatile platform for immuno-oncology and drug discovery. Oncoimmunology 8:e1670019, 2019.

74. J Kondo, T Ekawa, H Endo et al.: High-throughput screening in colorectal cancer tissue-originated spheroids. Cancer Sci. 110:345–355, 2019.

75. M Zanoni, M Cortesi, A Zamagni et al.: Modeling neoplastic disease with spheroids and organoids. J. Hematol. Oncol. 13:97, 2020.

76. F Foglietta, R Canaparo, G Muccioli et al.: Methodological aspects and pharmacological applications of three-dimensional cancer cell cultures and organoids. Life Sci. 254:117784, 2020.

77. F Weeber, M van de Wetering, M Hoogstraat et al.: Preserved genetic diversity in organoids cultured from biopsies of human colorectal cancer metastases. Proc. Natl. Acad. Sci. USA 112:13308–13311, 2015.

78. M van de Wetering, HE Francies, JM Francis et al.: Prospective derivation of a living organoid biobank of colorectal cancer patients. Cell 161:933–945, 2015.

79. Y Kiyohara, K Yoshino, S Kubota et al.: Drug screening and grouping by sensitivity with a panel of primary cultured cancer spheroids derived from endometrial cancer. Cancer Sci. 107:452–460, 2016.

80. J Kondo and M Inoue: Application of cancer organoid model for drug screening and personalized therapy. Cells 8:470, 2019.

81. T Liu, C Delavaux and YS Zhang: 3D bioprinting for oncology applications. J. 3D Print. Med. 3:55–58, 2019.

82. S Mao, Y Pang, T Liu et al.: Bioprinting of in vitro tumor models for personalized cancer treatment: A review. Biofabrication 12:042001, 2020.

83. EM Langer, BL Allen-Petersen, SM King et al.: Modeling tumor phenotypes in vitro with three-dimensional bioprinting. Cell Rep. 26:608–623.e6, 2019.

84. HG Yi, YH Jeong, Y Kim et al.: A bioprinted human-glioblastoma-on-a-chip for the identification of patient-specific responses to chemoradiotherapy. Nat. Biomed. Eng. 3:509–519, 2019.

85. Z Koledova: 3D cell culture: An introduction. Methods Mol. Biol. 1612:1–11, 2017.

86. S Knowlton, S Onal, CH Yu et al.: Bioprinting for cancer research. Trends Biotechnol. 33:504–513, 2015.

87. W Peng, P Datta, B Ayan et al.: 3D bioprinting for drug discovery and development in pharmaceutics. Acta Biomater. 57:26–46, 2017.

88. I Matai, G Kaur, A Seyedsalehi et al.: Progress in 3D bioprinting technology for tissue/organ regenerative engineering. Biomaterials 226:119536, 2020.

89. P Datta, M Dey, Z Ataie et al.: 3D bioprinting for reconstituting the cancer microenvironment. NPJ Precis. Oncol. 4:18, 2020.

90. G Rijal and W Li: A versatile 3D tissue matrix scaffold system for tumor modeling and drug screening. Sci. Adv. 3:e1700764, 2017.

91. MA Heinrich, R Bansal, T Lammers et al.: 3D-bioprinted mini-brain: A glioblastoma model to study cellular interactions and therapeutics. Adv. Mater. 31:e1806590, 2019.

92. S Mao, J He, Y Zhao et al.: Bioprinting of patient-derived in vitro intrahepatic cholangiocarcinoma tumor model: Establishment, evaluation and anti-cancer drug testing. Biofabrication 12:045014, 2020.

93. M Tang, Q Xie, RC Gimple et al.: Three-dimensional bioprinted glioblastoma microenvironments model cellular dependencies and immune interactions. Cell Res., 30:833–853, 2020.

94. Y Zhao, R Yao, L Ouyang et al.: Three-dimensional printing of Hela cells for cervical tumor model in vitro. Biofabrication 6:035001, 2014.

95. I Doh, YJ Kwon, B Ku et al.: Drug efficacy comparison of 3D forming and preforming sphere models with a micropillar and microwell chip platform. SLAS Discov. 24:476–483, 2019.

96. K Gorshkov, CZ Chen, RE Marshall et al.: Advancing precision medicine with personalized drug screening. Drug Discov. Today 24:272–278, 2019.

97. B Turanli, O Altay, J Boren et al.: Systems biology based drug repositioning for development of cancer therapy. Semin. Cancer Biol. 68:47–58, 2021.

98. P Nowak-Sliwinska, L Scapozza and IAA Ruiz: Drug repurposing in oncology: Compounds, pathways, phenotypes and computational approaches for colorectal cancer. Biochim. Biophys. Acta Rev. Cancer 1871:434–454, 2019.

99. GL Law, J Tisoncik-Go, MJ Korth et al.: Drug repurposing: A better approach for infectious disease drug discovery? Curr. Opin. Immunol. 25:588–592, 2013.

100. H Yuan, S Myers, J Wang et al.: Use of reprogrammed cells to identify therapy for respiratory papillomatosis. N. Engl. J. Med. 367: 1220–1227, 2012.

101. MJ Alvarez, Y Shen, FM Giorgi et al.: Functional characterization of somatic mutations in cancer using network-based inference of protein activity. Nat. Genet. 48:838–847, 2016.

102. MJ Alvarez, PS Subramaniam, LH Tang et al.: A precision oncology approach to the pharmacological targeting of mechanistic dependencies in neuroendocrine tumors. Nat. Genet. 50:979–989, 2018.

103. A Califano and MJ Alvarez: The recurrent architecture of tumour initiation, progression and drug sensitivity. Nat. Rev. Cancer 17:116–130, 2017.

104. R Khamsi: Computing cancer's weak spots. Science 368: 1174–1177, 2020.

105. A Chari, DT Vogl, M Gavriatopoulou et al.: Oral selinexor-dexamethasone for triple-class refractory multiple myeloma. N. Engl. J. Med. 381:727–738, 2019.

106. F Weeber, SN Ooft, KK Dijkstra et al.: Tumor organoids as a pre-clinical cancer model for drug discovery. Cell Chem. Biol. 24: 1092–1100, 2017.

107. Z Jia, Y Wang, L Cao et al.: First-line treatment selection with organoids of an EGFRm + TP53 m stage IA1 patient with early metastatic recurrence after radical surgery and follow-up. J. Thorac. Dis. 12: 3764–3773, 2020.

Cambridge Elements $\equiv$

Molecular Oncology

Edward P. Gelmann

University of Arizona

Dr. Edward P. Gelmann is John Norton Professor of Prostate Cancer Research at the University of Arizona and the University of Arizona Cancer Center. Dr. Gelmann previously headed Divisions of Hematology/Oncology at both Georgetown University and Columbia University. He has been the recipient of NIH, DOD and NIEHS grants for his research that has spanned cancer basic, clinical, and population sciences. Dr. Gelmann's research currently focuses on the early stages of prostate carcinogenesis and the development of novel therapeutics for prostate cancer. He continues to be involved in clinical care and clinical research of genitourinary malignancies. He has an active clinical practice and directs GU clinical research at the Cancer Center. Dr. Gelmann has published extensively and is senior editor of the book *Molecular Oncology: Causes of Cancer and Targets for Treatment* (Cambridge University Press, 2013).

About the Series

Therapeutics in clinical oncology are based increasingly on molecular drivers and hallmarks of cancers. *Elements in Molecular Oncology* provides a timely overview of topics in oncology for researchers and clinicians. By focusing on cancer sites or pathways, this series presents information on the latest findings on cancer causation and treatment.

Cambridge Elements ≡

Molecular Oncology

Elements in the Series

Personalized Drug Screening for Functional Tumor Profiling
Victoria El-Khoury, Tatiana Michel, Hichul Kim, and Yong-Jun Kwon

A full series listing is available at: www.cambridge.org/EMO

Printed in the United States
by Baker & Taylor Publisher Services

Printed in the United States
by Baker & Taylor Publisher Services